The Booby Trap

Bust Out Of Breast Cancer And Heal Yourself

Heidi Sorensen

Copyright 2022 By Heidi Sorensen

Author's Legal Disclaimer

This book is solely for educational and informational purposes and is not medical advice. It is not intended as a substitute for the medical advice of physicians. The reader should regularly consult a medical professional in matters relating to his/her health, and particularly concerning any symptoms that may require medical diagnosis or attention.

Any use of the information within this book is at the reader's discretion and risk. The author cannot be held responsible for any loss, claim, or damage arising out of the use, or misuse, of information within this book, or the failure to take medical advice.

No part of this publication may be reproduced, transmitted, or sold in any form without the prior written consent of the author, except in the case of brief quotations as part of reviews and certain other non-commercial uses permitted by copyright law.

This book is dedicated to my beautiful mother — the most resilient and courageous woman I know.

Contents

Introduction	vii

Part One
My Story

1. From Giving Life To Fearing Death	3
2. 'Just In Case'	8

Part Two
Healing Naturally

3. Step 1	19
4. Step 2	31
5. Step 3	36
6. Step 4	44
7. Step 5	53
8. Step 6	62

Part Three
Nutrition For The Body, Mind & Soul

9. The Happy Healing Project	69
10. Eat To Stop Cancer Diet	78
Afterword	83
About the Author	87

Introduction

Now that you've picked up *The Booby Trap,* I'm guessing that you're someone who's searching for effective holistic approaches to dealing with, or preventing, breast cancer. Let's face it, when diagnosed, there are a lot of decisions to make and factors to consider and everything happens fast.

I know how overwhelming it can be — because I've walked the same path as you. If you are anything like I was, you want the best possible tools in your tool belt to help you through it. This book is for those who want to take the bull by the horns and do a deeper dive into holistic mind-set healing.

Are you passionate in your search for answers? Do you want more information than what western medicine offers and instinctively know that there is more than one way to heal from breast cancer? And do you yearn to heal mentally, physically, and spiritually because you understand this is the only way to truly get well?

This could mean that you've decided to forgo traditional methods, or it could just mean you want to add holistic practices into your current protocol. Either way is great.

In this book, I'm going to share with you a system of powerful natural healing methods that I discovered on my journey to banish cancer. You'll learn how a specific combination of holistic practices helped me recover my health in the fastest way possible. You can access them all too. I'm here to lend a hand, offer some helpful advice, and demonstrate what's possible.

But why listen to me? My name is Heidi Sorensen and I was 37 years old and had just given birth to a beautiful baby girl when I was diagnosed with breast cancer. I was warned by doctors that I would die if I chose to go down a natural healing route.

That was 25 years ago.

Today, I'm a counselor and health mentor for women with breast cancer and other health-related issues. I'm also a certified mindfulness meditation teacher, a public speaker on using our mindset for healing, and have been practicing Kriya Yoga meditation for over four decades. I'm also very passionate about advocating for the rights of girls and women and have worked with some amazing organizations including, The Ending Violence Association of Canada and the United States Department of Defense on an international project supporting women.

You may be wondering — what is 'The Booby Trap'? The title has a few meanings for me. First, it represents the potential trap of falling into the western medical system's cancer 'box' and getting stuck without directions on how to get out. This box works well for some people, but not for all. The western system prescribes a protocol that is standard — chemotherapy, radiation and pharmaceutical drugs. They don't seem to like it much when we ask about other options or tell them we want to explore other methods. They prefer to keep us in their box because it is all they are taught in medical school and they can control the dialogue and structure around the contents of that box. Inside this box is the rules and regulations of what they prescribe when you get breast cancer.

In The Booby Trap, I reflect on my experiences with doctors trying to get me in the box and explain why I refused. I tell my story and the many challenges that confronted me along the way by people who doubted my choices and a medical system that was not designed for people who thought the way I did. I knew they had good intentions, but their ideas didn't align with mine.

What if we want to do something else alongside the standard western protocol, or instead of? We shouldn't be dismissed or considered 'woo-woo' if we want to incorporate holistic healing choices into our journey. We need to be heard and respected and not ridiculed because of our questions or opinions. Our breasts and our bodies are dynamic. They are in a constant state of change and recalibration and have an innate intelligence towards achieving a healthy and balanced state. Holistic practices can nurture this intelligence and make the healthy state happen quicker for us.

We can also get caught in the booby trap of the opinions of the people around us. Well-meaning family members and friends all believe they have the right solution for you. But, because fear is the dominant emotion when we are diagnosed with breast cancer, our loved ones are usually speaking from a place of fear. And since we are also afraid, we can be more susceptible to being talked into things that don't resonate with us. After speaking with doctors, family and friends, we may become confused, intimidated, or feel as though our thoughts and feelings about our health don't really matter. I'm here to tell you — they do!

The booby trap also refers to our own way of thinking. If not mindful, we can fall prey to fear and negativity during our illness and stay in this space, effectively relinquishing our participation in our healing process. As humans, most of us have a limited perception of what we are capable of in respect to healing ourselves. It can be easy to feel powerless and fall into to the victim space when confronted by disease, but this can be a dangerous place to stay in for too long.

One of my primary goals in writing this book is to emphasize why it is so important to take an active role in your healing process. By accepting responsibility for your health, you have consciously sparked the healing fire inside of you to begin its work.

In my early, adult years I was very much living a dual life. I was a model, actor and singer, working in various countries around the globe. I was also a Playboy centerfold, navigating the tricky world of celebrity and Hollywood superficiality. Like many women, I have seen first-hand the impact of a patriarchal society and its effects on women and their self-esteem. In the midst of it all, something tragic happened that would affect the course of my life — the brutal murder of a friend at the hands of her husband. To see a kind, beautiful 20 year old woman with such a promising future ahead of her destroyed in a fit of jealousy and violence was almost more than I could bare. It was during this difficult period that I began to discover my true voice. It became easy, necessary even, to speak up when I saw other young women experiencing injustices around me.

After her death, I felt I had no choice but to stand up against the inequities that I was witnessing. I began to notice that the words I used had some power, that people would often listen and that I had the capacity to affect change.

These early experiences became the catalyst that sparked my passion for advocating for the rights of women, including their right to live a healthy life, free of disease. I began working alongside various government and non-government organizations and charities around the world, including my own non-profit society for girls and women which allowed me to bear witness to many of the health struggles girls and women face on a daily basis.

Although women make up 50 percent of the world population, there is a vast history of gender bias which is widespread in healthcare systems around the globe, and yes, even in North America. Studies show that stereotypes about gender affect how doctors treat illnesses and approach their patients, including how much time is given to patients to explain their diagnosis. Not surprisingly, women get significantly less time in the doctor's office. It's no accident that the word 'uterus' originates from the word 'hysteria.' There is still a pervasive belief in the medical community that anytime a woman complains about her health it's either related to her hormones or it's all in her head.

Initially, I was given a false negative breast cancer diagnosis by a doctor who claimed the lump in my breast was from nursing my baby. This mishap caused a several month delay in my cancer diagnosis and as we all know cancer grows fast and time is always of the essence.

Because I had done mental rehearsal before with meditation to help change various conditions in my life, it only made sense to tap into this quantum field of unlimited potential to help heal myself when I got breast cancer. The quantum field is one of the names given to the space where you can change the current 'sick' energetic version of you into a healthy, cancer free version of you by doing what is called 'mental rehearsal,' or imagining and feeling that you are completely well. This information has been available for thousands of years and documented by various spiritual saints and masters. In the current era, Dr. Joe Dispenza, author of many inspiring books including, 'Becoming Supernatural,' is proving the science behind 'changing matter' inside our bodies.

I am offering my own unique, guided meditations specifically designed for breast cancer to access and bring into form, the perfect, healthy version of you. You can find these meditations on my website at www.holisticbreastexpert.com.

We are not victims of circumstance. Things don't happen to us. We create our lives, intentionally. We attract what we think and believe. Somewhere along the way, we got out of alignment with our emotional health and have created dis-ease. We are also capable of getting back into alignment and creating perfect health!

In the upcoming chapters, I discuss the importance of our thoughts and words during and after breast cancer. We can be our own worst enemy when we constantly think and speak about the disease we are facing and our runaway, fearful thoughts can do more harm than we know.

You are only a victim of breast cancer if you believe you are. The Booby Trap offers strategies to help laser focus your mindset to perfect health.

You will learn:

- How to take charge of your healing process and minimize emotional suffering.
- That your thoughts and words you use during your illness have immense power and can affect your recovery.
- Why 'remission' and 'survivor' may not be the best choice of words to use to identify yourself.
- How to gain control of your thoughts and words quickly for a more positive, health outcome.
- Why emotional wounds being held in your body system may be blocking you from living a healthy life.
- Practical ways to address these emotional wounds for deep healing.
- What nutritious and holistic remedies I used to powerfully cleanse and nourish my body, preventing cancer from thriving in my system.

The biggest reason I wrote this book was so I could be of service to women. Breast cancer can be very intimidating and confusing. When I had breast cancer, I searched for a mentor to guide and inspire me. I was looking for an individual who had been there and done that — but I couldn't find anyone. There were also very few books written by women who had forged their own holistic path that had the advice that I desperately needed. I'm hoping *The Booby Trap* can be that book for you.

It is my sincere wish that my words offer the wisdom of someone who has been through the fire and come out the other side. Remember, change *can* happen in a day — don't let anyone tell you otherwise. Just now, 100,000 chemical reactions are taking place in every single one of your cells. If you multiply 100,000 chemical reactions by the 100 trillion cells in your body — the answer is a mind-boggling number of chemical reactions that are happening inside you, every second. Change is occurring inside your body constantly whether you like it or not — so why not participate and be an active partner with it, to change it for the better? Be patient and kind to yourself as you navigate your journey. You deserve this self-love because you are a magnificent being with a divine purpose on this earth.

Don't wait to get started. Every day counts. The tips and strategies you are about to learn have proven results. Each chapter provides new secrets that will help you stay in control of your journey. Practice the principles I've outlined in this book and you will emerge from your breast cancer experience happier, healthier and feeling more alive than ever before.

You will be proud of yourself.

You will feel empowered because you took an active role in your journey.

You will have learned invaluable mindset skills that can benefit you in all areas of your life.

You will have a better, more inspiring story, void of victimhood.

You will not identify as a survivor, but as a conqueror.

You will tell others how you tapped into the power that creates all life and used that power to create a happier and more vital version of you. Then, *you* may write a book or tell your story and be an inspiration to others — and so it goes.

Breast cancer shook up my life — for the better. It challenged me, but in a good way. It heightened the happiness factor in my life and made me feel more present. It made me stronger, more resilient, more grateful, and more aligned with my higher power. I try not to take things for granted and I pay more attention to the subtle moments of my day.

This is my highest desire for you, dear one. As humans, we are all connected and as women, even more so. Your journey is also my journey. I love you and bow to you for your courage and determination. I honor you and send all my love, peace and prayers to you to live a magnificent, happy and healthy life.

Part One

My Story

Chapter 1

From Giving Life To Fearing Death

"Everything is energy, and that's all there is to it. Match the healing frequencies of the reality you want, and you cannot help but get that reality. There can be no other way. This is no philosophy; this is physics" – Albert Einstein.

At 37 years old, right after the birth of my daughter, I was told I had breast cancer. It quickly became the best and worst year of my life. My question was — how on earth could this happen to someone like me?

By all standards, I was young and very healthy. I ate extremely well and exercised every day. I was super into juicing and cleansing. I took herbs and vitamins, didn't smoke and very rarely drank alcohol. In fact, I was the woman that all my friends came to for advice on health issues. If they wanted to know how to get glowing skin, or lose a few pounds, I had the solution. If they wanted natural remedies for any minor ailment, I knew what to do. I was very much into natural remedies and a walking testimony for good health.

Or so I thought.

When I got breast cancer, it was an absolute shock. I was young and a new mother and the diagnosis came out of left field. As with any serious diagnosis, we don't want to believe it's true. There's something strange about being in your thirties and being told you have cancer. It's surreal.

I will never know exactly why I got breast cancer, but I have some ideas. Under the surface, I was very anxious about my life. My marriage wasn't going well and finances were shaky, at best. My husband and I had just come through a turbulent time living in Los Angeles, with the riots and the Northridge earthquake and our lives were very much in flux.

What I didn't realize at the time was I also had unresolved pain and unforgiveness towards my father that needed to be worked out. I eventually began to learn that trapped emotions in our bodies can play a critical role in disease developing.

Then I got pregnant. I couldn't imagine the chaos we were living in with a baby. I started to panic and with a marriage that was already under stress, I knew I either had to move back to Canada where my family was or find a safe place away from the city that would allow me some peace while I was pregnant.

I looked up and down the coast of Los Angeles trying to find a nook of a place to live that offered clean air and a laid-back lifestyle that would be good to raise a child in, but all the rentals were so expensive and I was losing hope. Then I found a little condo in Malibu that I thought would work financially so I packed everything up and moved to Malibu. My husband was off in Europe shooting a documentary and so at seven months pregnant and with the strength of my Viking ancestors I moved all of our belongings to Malibu.

I suppose I may have been fuelled by some sort of

strength that pregnant women get when under the gun to nest. The craziness of the L.A. riots were fresh in my mind. The memories of people running through our yard with AK47's strapped to their backs, jumping our fences. At the height of the riot we decided to leave our home and backing down our driveway we found our local Korean grocery store up in flames. After the riots I found myself sitting on my bed, rocking back and forth, crying. I was stressed to the core.

Moving to Malibu turned out to be a good decision. I was starting to unwind and enjoy my pregnancy. There were lots of long walks on the beach and I was beginning to make friends. Things were looking up. I even got a writing break and was asked to write a project for a well-known A list actor.

Soon, I gave birth to a beautiful baby girl. And then, I found the little lump. It was the same lump that I felt right before I got pregnant and ignored because who would think that a 36 year old healthy woman would have breast cancer? Seriously, so ridiculous!

The swelling in my breasts went down after the pregnancy and suddenly that little lump that I had ignored, reappeared. Oh right, forgot about that. I was busy growing a baby, so it kind of left my mind.

I found 'the best' radiologist in Los Angeles only to have him tell me that I had a clogged milk duct due to the pregnancy. When I tried to tell him I had the lump before I got pregnant, he scoffed. He said: "go home, you're fine". A few months later, I noticed the lump was a bit bigger, so off I went again to see the same doctor. This time, he confirmed it was cancer. The false negative diagnosis he had given me months before had cost me precious time.

I didn't believe the diagnosis at first because it didn't

make any sense to me. I was a brand new mother. All of my focus for the last several months had been centered around my pregnancy and giving birth to my child. Within moments I had been robbed of the bliss that every mother experiences when having a baby and enjoying the first year of life with her. I was now in fight or flight mode. I was in a fight for survival, not only for myself but for my daughter who I was determined to not leave motherless.

What would I do? Would I blindly go down the path of western conventional medicine that everyone goes down? It felt overwhelming to me not to come from a place of knowledge before I met with doctors. I immediately started researching the type of breast cancer that I had.

I knew I needed to get educated so I could make the right healing decision for myself. I didn't know exactly what I was going to do, but I knew I was on an intense time limit to figure it out. The surgery was being scheduled and options were being discussed already and the pressure was on. I immersed myself in books on the subject of breast cancer.

Then I received more devastating news. Because I was nursing my baby, the doctor told me I needed to stop immediately so I could have the surgery. No doctor would operate on a breast that was full of milk. In fact, he recommended drugs to dry up the milk ducts quickly. I was floored.

There I was, a young woman who had just given birth, nursing my new baby daughter and then told to stop immediately to have life-saving surgery. Naturally, I was devastated.

After doing some research, I ended up refusing the drug. It just didn't feel right to me. I compromised with my doctor and continued to nurse my baby on my left breast and let the right one dry up naturally. This wasn't the solution my doctor was looking for, but he had no choice but to listen to me. So, my baby continued to nurse on my left breast and we abandoned the right one to do its thing and dry up. It took a week or two more than the drugs would have, but it was worth it to me.

By the time the surgery date came around, there was still a little bit of milk left in the ducts and the surgeon didn't feel comfortable operating on it. So, I found a different surgeon and by the time the surgery date was set, the milk had mostly dried up. Fortunately, the surgery was a success.

Maybe it was a bit risky to take the time to let the milk dry up naturally — I don't know. But, the choice had been mine and I felt good about it. And it worked. I was a new mother and nursing my baby was important to me. I did it my way in my own time and played a part in my healing journey. I listened to the experts and then figured out a plan that worked for me.

Chapter 2

'Just In Case'

Now that the lump was out, I had to continue with the research and learn more about the type of cancer I had and what would be the best healing option for me. Someone recommended a top oncologist in Los Angeles, so off I went. I walked into her ultra-chic, office on the most expensive real estate in the heart of Beverly Hills.

The oncologist seemed nice enough sitting behind her desk in her posh office. I quickly noticed her designer jacket and shoes as I sat down across from her. She looked up from her paperwork and spent very little time getting to the point. She said she had studied my file and was recommending chemotherapy and radiation. She was also recommending the drug tomoxefen to help curb the estrogen which she said would put me into early menopause. I blinked. Was she kidding? She wasn't. In fact, there was nothing funny going on in that office.

It took the oncologist less than a minute to deliver that news.

I took a deep breath. I had been doing a lot of research on the subject of my particular type of breast cancer and discovered some interesting facts. I told her that according to my research there was no evidence that chemotherapy worked for my particular type of breast cancer and asked her why she would recommend it to me.

I'll never forget the look on her face for as long as I live. It was a mix of surprise that I knew that information combined with a faint glimpse of the 'caught in the act' look. In that moment — I had my answer.

She took a second and then responded with these exact words that I also shall never forget. *"You are correct; there is no evidence that chemotherapy is effective for your type of cancer."*

So I asked her the obvious question: "Then why are you recommending it to me?" Another long pause. She could tell that I wasn't going to leave until I got her to admit the truth and what she said I know was the truth. I could see it in the shift of her expression.

She said: "Because by law, I have to recommend chemotherapy to you, just in case."

I was shocked. We stared at each other awkwardly. Then I said, "In case what?" And she replied: "In case it works." But, what I heard was, "I have to recommend it to you in case you come back and sue me." The United States was a mecca for medical lawsuits — this I knew.

When faced with a life-threatening illness and you are talking to the person who is supposed to be 'saving you,' it's hard to say no thank you, I don't totally trust that you can actually save me. It's a bit like drowning in the ocean and a boat comes by that's leaking profusely and the well-meaning captain offers you a hand. You think, maybe there's another option — like a sturdy log that's floating by. Maybe it's a better idea to jump on that log and paddle back to shore. It might seem risky to tell the captain no, but if our intuition is telling us to say no, then shouldn't we trust it? All I knew was, I wasn't going to just say yes to something that felt so wrong.

Just in case.

I had read all about chemotherapy and I knew the incredible havoc it creates in our bodies. I understood that more people die from the effects of chemotherapy than the actual cancer. And if there was no evidence saying it worked for my type of breast cancer, why on earth would I take it? Destroy all my healthy cells, lose my hair, go into menopause at 37 years old and become weak and immune compromised — *just in case?*

If there had been overwhelming evidence stating that chemo helped my type of breast cancer then perhaps I would have considered it. But, there wasn't.

So as I looked at the Beverly Hills oncologist with the blue Prada shoes something came over me and my body just sort of stood up. I remember distinctly just standing there wondering why I had stood up. It was as if a force greater than myself had just pushed me out of the chair and said:

"Get up Heidi and walk out the door." That's what I heard in my head: *"Get up and get out."*

So I said to the doctor: "No thank you. I'm going to pass, but thank you for your time." and walked out.

My mother taught me to think for myself, to question authority and do what feels right for me. I didn't want to be part of a system of patients who blindly give away their power because they are afraid. We get diagnosed with a life-threatening disease like cancer and we are horribly afraid it makes it hard to think properly so we do whatever the first doctor that comes along tells us to do. It's a trap that we are all very susceptible to falling into.

Fear makes us freeze — until we catch our breath and

find the ability to stop everything and listen to our intuition instead of our 'fear voice.' Without a doubt, I was more afraid of the chemotherapy than the cancer.

Also, I didn't like that everything was so fancy in this doctor's Beverly Hills office. It was apparent that the business of cancer was a big business. I didn't need a Beverly Hills office with a posh doctor wearing designer shoes to convince me to take chemo. I needed EVIDENCE. And there was none.

Also, I didn't want to contribute to this oncologist's designer wardrobe. I mean, I liked it. I just didn't want to help *pay for it*. I wanted to feel good about my choice of healing and one thing I knew for sure was that this didn't feel good and I needed more time to think.

I didn't know it at the time, but I was hard core listening to my intuition and being led by a guiding force much bigger than myself. Interestingly, when I walked out, she didn't say a word. I decided to get another opinion from a different oncologist. The other top oncologist in town. Unfortunately, this fellow couldn't make eye contact and had the bed side manner of a cardboard box. He advised the same protocol as the first oncologist; chemo, radiation and tomoxefen. Once again, his recommendation took under a minute. Surely there had to be an alternative to this archaic protocol. I asked him if there were any other alternatives and he quickly said there was not.

Once again, I felt my body stand up.

My husband gave me an "already?" look and I nodded. It was time to go. I told the doctor that I wasn't going to do chemo because there was no evidence showing that chemo worked for my type of breast cancer — the exact same conversation I'd just had with the Prada oncologist. But, instead of giving me the same "Yes, you're right" look that she had, this guy actually said: "If you don't do what I am recommending for you, you will die."

Die. That's what he said.

Now, you may be thinking, what's up with Heidi? Why is she surrounded by doctors that are pissing her off? Maybe it's her. Maybe she's the one with the problem. And you might be right. I did have a problem and my problem was that I didn't like being told that I was going to die unless I did what a doctor told me to do. He was playing God but he had forgotten one thing — that he actually wasn't God.

How did he know I would die? Was he sure? Why would he tell me that unless he was absolutely sure?

My hands started to shake and, as long as I live, I will never forget the walk from his office to the outside of the building. It was the longest, short walk I've ever had. With my baby in my arms, I stumbled down the hallway, dizzy with confusion and shock. I passed the receptionist who looked up at me with concern. I was trying in vain to hold in the tears, but they came anyway.

The people in the waiting room stared at me, felt sorry for me and most likely thought I was dying too. I didn't know if my husband was following me out or not until I got to the door and I heard his voice yelling at the doctor: "Who the f*** do you think you are — God?"

When we got home, my husband called the doctor's office and told the receptionist that if we didn't get an apology letter signed by him by the next day, we would sue him for emotional distress. The next day a Fed-X truck rolled up and the carrier hand delivered an apology letter signed by the doctor.

We felt somewhat vindicated, I suppose. But I still needed to do something about the breast cancer. I was tired of going up against doctors that had a single-minded focus and had no additional healing protocols to offer me besides chemo and radiation. I knew it wasn't their fault; these were all the tools they had ever been given.

After I said no to both oncologists, I was a little lost and quite frankly, a bit scared. What had I done?

After the dust settled, I realized one very important thing. And this was the lesson for me in all the chaos. I had stood up for myself and listened to my inner voice and didn't turn over my power to just any doctor. I would wait for the right doctor that resonated with me, a doctor that I liked and that I trusted. Because picking a doctor is very much like picking a best friend. You look for certain qualities that you can rely on. You need to like them, trust them, respect them and believe in them. You need to have *rapport*.

I know every breast cancer diagnosis is unique and I felt like I was doing what was right for my particular case. I know that some women don't have a choice and if the results of my research for my case had been different then I may have had to do chemo and radiation in order to save my life. But, this wasn't the case, so I kept searching. I knew there were other options.

I've always been a very spiritual person and my feeling is that whatever happens to us in our life time happens for a reason. I understood that this illness had meaning and even though I didn't know what that meaning was yet, I felt I had to stay close to my higher power in order to get through it in one piece. I was already bucking the system pretty hard and I needed strength. So, I prayed and asked God to present the right path for me.

Meanwhile, I was getting pushback. People were calling me, trying to be helpful and pushing me to do the chemo. Luckily, my husband was behind me one hundred percent.

He understood that he had to step out of my way and that whatever I decided to do had to be my decision.

To make things worse, because I wasn't taking quick action, my best friend had become convinced that I was in denial. She wrote me a long letter stating how worried she was because I was saying no to all the doctors and she felt I was not only putting my life in danger but also my baby's life. It was a very passive aggressive letter, basically telling me I was wrong for what I was doing. I was devastated. I felt alone and even more scared.

The words from my friend crushed me. Little did she know I was in the opposite of denial. I was taking a very pro-active, if not aggressive, stance in my healing process. I was a research queen. I knew what I was doing. I felt shock, betrayal, anger, disappointment, sadness, overwhelm, and many other crazy emotions as I read the letter at stop lights while driving down the Pacific Coast Highway. I pulled over and cried my eyes out.

I hated her in that moment for not understanding me. But, I knew she was just scared. I also knew that her opinions were in the majority. She would have been one of those people who would have just done what the doctors said. She would have thanked them and not threatened to sue them for being arrogant. She would have found their static opinions helpful in some way. Why couldn't I be like that? It would have been easier. I didn't necessarily enjoy bucking the system. I didn't have some need to be a rebel.

Yet there I was, *becoming one.*

I needed to find a way forward. I sat on the side of the highway with her letter in my hand and I prayed while my baby slept in the back. A cop came by on his motorcycle and tapped on my window. I must have looked like a crazy woman with the tears. He asked me if I was okay and I said yes but he knew I wasn't. I told him I didn't need any help, but I knew that I did, just not the kind of help he could offer. I felt truly alone in the world.

After he left, I sat there for a few more minutes and prayed. I prayed for answers and for strength. I prayed for a way forward that I could feel good about. Then, I opened my eyes and found the strength inside myself to carry on with my day. I decided right then and there to turn my power over to God to guide me and protect me. I needed to trust and have faith that I would overcome this challenge.

Soon after, things started to shift. I was introduced to a doctor who I resonated with and trusted. It was the beginning and I was so happy and grateful that I had waited, tuned out the doubters and listened to my intuition.

Part Two

Healing Naturally

Chapter 3

Step 1

Shifting Out Of Fear

"When fear disappears, the foundation of disease is gone."
— *A Course in Miracles.*

The cure rates for cancer today are high, depending on the tumor type, the stage and grade of the tumor, and how aggressive the cancer is. Even if it isn't cured, cancer can often become a chronic disease today (like diabetes or high blood pressure). So why is the fear of cancer so great? It's a habit from the past century when a diagnosis of cancer was a death sentence. Don S. Dizon, MD, Clinical Co-Director at Massachusetts General Hospital Cancer Center, says: "Cancer does not equal death. That's what we need to tell people. Among the first things I tell patients facing a new diagnosis is: "you're not dying."

Ninety-five percent of breast cancers are cured when caught early. So there is no reason to be 'scared to death.' When we take a pro-active stance in our healing process the fear of the disease will turn to gratefulness. Grateful that we have been given the opportunity to learn how to heal ourselves and find deeper meaning in our lives.

But, fear seems to have a life of its own.

My breast cancer diagnosis came out of left field. I was young and healthy and had just given birth to my baby. It shocked and scared the hell out of me. I had no words — only tears. I stepped into massive fear, immediately.

As humans we are hard-wired to think about the worst case scenario when confronted with difficult situations, especially disease. This is the primitive brain that when faced with potential danger triggers the fight or flight response. It is meant to help us. But, often it's fear on over drive. We need to work diligently to keep that primitive brain in check because fear isn't always rational. After all, its acronym is *false evidence appearing real*.

The more we stay in the state of fear, the more our brains and bodies work to hold us in the 'fight or flight' mode. This state takes away from our body's natural healing resources, directing energy for combat or defence against whatever threat is coming.

When you get cancer, you get scared — scared of suffering, scared of dying and losing everything and everyone you love. Some people get so scared that they can't even think properly. They are in heightened and prolonged fight or flight mode and prolonged fear disconnects you completely from your healing power.

Fear can feel like a tangible entity that enters our beings — it is a very uncomfortable, physical feeling. I had an intuition about the direction I wanted to go with my healing but I didn't know how to get there because the fear was so great and was clouding my judgement. But, at least I figured out what direction I *didn't* want to go in — and that helped steer me.

Being a rebel in a system of medical obedience isn't easy. However, I was up for the challenge. I was ready for anything that came my way. I felt deeply that I needed a bit more information and a bit more time. Against the advice of the doctors I decided to take a few more days to figure out what I needed to do. I also desperately needed some time to stop the madness — this massive fear and uncertainty that I had become entrapped in.

I knew if I could just step outside of the fear vortex that I could think more clearly and make better decisions for my health. I knew I had to lift my energetic frequency to a place that would allow me to heal and that staying in the fear zone was a dangerous place to be. I had to find a way to calibrate to the highest energy level I could, which involved changing my thoughts and my entire mind-set. Dr. Wayne Dyer said it well.

> *"...When you bring a higher and a more loving energy to the presence of disorder or disharmony or disease, you are really bringing a healing energy. And that's what healing is involved with: It's no longer allowing yourself to wallow around in a process in which you tell yourself that you don't have the capacity to be able to transcend whatever it is that's bothering you or hurting you or killing you."*

My intuition was telling me very strongly to research more holistic approaches since I had now discovered that chemotherapy wasn't effective for the type of breast cancer that I had. Yet, everyone around me was operating at such a high pitch level of urgency that I found it hard to find mental silence so I could think. I needed to stop the roller-coaster. So I pulled on the emergency brake and stopped talking to the negative chatterers in my life.

A family member was calling me, telling me I should

listen to the doctors and do as they said. I loved her but I felt she was interfering with the plan I was putting together for myself and it was causing even more stress and fear. I started avoiding her calls. Despite her good intentions, her persistence wasn't helping.

Next, I stopped talking to my best friend temporarily because in this moment she wasn't helping either. My family member and friend were trapped in the fear zone and because of that, they wanted me to surrender to whatever the doctors told me to do. This is a common occurrence, especially for women. Fear immobilizes us so we simply turn over our power.

I am not opposed to following advice from doctors. I value their opinions and honor the dedicated work that they do. I just know that I have opinions too and I may need to ask a lot of questions before I am satisfied. It's my body and whether it's cancer or any other issue, I always want to consider a variety of options and most importantly, a say in how I heal my body.

A woman's intuition can be a very clear guiding light, if we pay attention to it. I was getting a very strong signal from my intuition that there was a better, more holistic way to heal. And if I was patient just a little bit longer, it would reveal itself. I can't explain this feeling. I just knew.

The tricky part of honoring our intuition is we don't always know what it is trying to tell us and sometimes we get it confused with fear. Knowing the difference between intuition and fear is very important especially if we are facing a life-threatening disease. We are getting bombarded with opinions that are scary and very real, so how on earth are we supposed to know how to listen to the still, small voice of intuition?

Intuition is often a knowing that is based on more

elements than the rational mind can deal with at any given moment.

You might say intuition is a subconscious assessment of a variety of elements:

- The past (experiences, knowledge),
- Personal needs and preferences (how do I want to feel) and
- The present (feelings that arise, choice of words, surroundings and signs other people are giving)

All of this leads to a conclusion of the best way to handle any given situation.

Oddly, fear and intuition are easily confused and this is because they are both experienced as a feeling that we get in our guts. Many of us have fallen out of touch with our gut feelings, to put it mildly. We're so occupied with our thoughts and intelligent reasoning, that it's hard to understand what our gut is telling us.

The two most important things that separate fear from intuition are:

Intuition is only about the present moment. Intuition is neutral and unemotional, whereas fear is highly emotionally charged. Reliable intuition feels right, it has a compassionate tone to it. It confirms that you are doing the right thing, without having an overly positive or negative tone.

Fear is often anxious, dark and heavy. It sometimes feels cruel or delusional. There is a feeling of stress and concern about the future.

I didn't know it at the time but I was creating a path for myself that was being guided by my very sacred intuition. So where does intuition ultimately come from? Intuition comes from the universal source energy or God — or whatever you prefer to call it.

There is overwhelming evidence that it is important to feel all your feelings and emotions, especially after a shocking diagnosis like cancer. The fear is so tangible it almost has a life of its own. We feel as though we have no control over it. It's heavy and dark and seems to come in waves whenever it damn well feels like it. So we know we can't just suddenly think rosy thoughts when we get cancer. We need to process. This takes a bit of time and it's different for everyone.

We need to feel all of the hard emotions because if we don't, they will most likely arise later on and cause more havoc than they would have initially. We need to grieve through our shock and fear before we can go forward. We can't suppress what we feel because there is no suppressing lava that wants to explode from the volcano. You can't put a lid on it. It will bubble and boil until the lid is blown off and the lava flows.

Sometimes, on the way to visit my doctor, I would cry. Driving down the Pacific Coast Highway, I would gaze out at the ocean and wonder the usual, 'why me' thoughts. I'm young and I *thought* I was healthy. I haven't been a bad person. I have never smoked and never drank much at all. So why me? It made me angry and confused. I also wondered why this would happen right after the birth of my daughter. It was like a cruel joke. My baby didn't deserve to have a sick mother facing a life-threatening illness. It all felt so wrong and I couldn't help but feel angry. I desperately needed to process these emotions.

After the tears, I would once again end up at my doctor's office for my usual holistic treatments and a dose of his silly jokes and happy attitude. I cherished the moments when I was with him because he truly believed I was going to be just fine. He would scientifically explain to me what he was doing and why it worked and it all made sense to me. I was in the right place for me.

The first step to overcoming fear is to become aware of it. To really take a good look at it. Take a moment to settle and breathe and then be present with the energy around the feeling. Witness the fear and breathe it out. Then, ask yourself what thoughts you are thinking that's creating the fear. Is it the fear that you won't get well and that you'll die? Understand that our imaginations create much scarier scenarios than what the actual truth is.

I had fearful thoughts and images of dying and leaving my baby motherless and countless other horrible scenarios that played out because of this false vision of my future. When we are immersed in fear, we can't tell the difference between what is actually happening and the thoughts we tell ourselves about the circumstance.

When we do this sort of imagining, we are projecting images of made-up events that have not happened and most likely will ever happen. Our minds want to take us to the absolute worst case scenario and then ruminate on that, over and over again. However, the fact is the survival rate for women with breast cancer has increased immensely and most women are getting well, with a much smaller percentage who aren't.

When you are caught in paralyzing fear, a good technique is the 4-7-8 method. The 4-7-8 method of breathing to calm the mind and body has its ancient roots in the yogic practice of pranayama, but was popularized by Dr. Andrew Weil in 2015. I used this technique when I felt my fear level rising to the point of it affecting my breath. We can't always just sit down and meditate for 20 minutes or longer when we are feeling panicky. Sometimes, we need a "right now" technique that helps us settle down and get to a better place.

The 4-7-8 Method

Steps:
Inhale through your nose for four counts.
Hold your breath for seven counts
Exhale through your nose for eight counts

Integrative medicine expert, Melissa Young, MD, states: "Yoga breathing techniques calm the body down and bring it into a more relaxed state. This kind of breathing can help us focus our mind and our body away from worries and repetitive thoughts." The counting process distracts our racing mind to the task, keeping it preoccupied.

The late Buddhist monk Thích Nhất Hạnh wrote: "Breathing in, I calm body and mind. Breathing out, I smile. Dwelling in the present moment, I know this is the only moment."

Nothing bad is ever happening in the present moment. It is only the past and the false future we create in our minds that hold us hostage.

The fear and grief of getting cancer doesn't have to remain debilitating. We are the creators of our thoughts. We are the creators of our lives. We get to choose how we want to handle our healing process. We can't let the fear speak for us and take charge of how things will play out.

I knew that my body had the power to heal without harsh chemicals, but at some point in time most of western society turned their power over to the pharmaceutical industry and because of this, I was considered the person who was making a strange choice for myself. I wasn't following the crowd. I wasn't operating the way I was supposed to — and that made people uncomfortable.

Medical doctors are not taught anything alternative in medical school, nor are they taught even one class in diet and nutrition. We have lots of choices. We have the power with our informed minds and strong intuition to work with our doctors and pick what is right for our bodies. But with the burden of fear impeding us, things get scary and much more difficult to navigate.

One of the most powerful tools we have is the ability to observe our thoughts and feelings. When a fearful thought arises, we need to stop it and bear witness to it. Like a cop telling the bad guy to stop in his tracks. Freeze! Just the simple act of becoming aware of our thought is a huge step. Here is the best part; once we observe our fear we immediately become separate from it. It is no longer a part of us. Suddenly, we are the witness of it; observing it. Once this happens, we become separate from it.

We need to go back into our lives and take inventory. Did you experience any trauma or difficult situations with family or loved ones? Were you abused or neglected? How did you process those events? Were you able to talk about it with anyone or did you suppress it? Were you afraid? Anything that wasn't processed is still sitting below the surface in what spiritual teacher and author of The power of Now, Eckhart Tolle likes to call the 'pain-body.'

Tolle describes the pain-body as an entity of its own. It is an accumulation of painful life experiences that was not fully faced and accepted in the moment it arose. Those experiences leave behind an energy residue of emotional pain and come together with other energy forms from other painful moments. After some time you have a pain-body —

an energy entity consisting of stuck, difficult emotions. Tolle asks us to be a witness to the pain that has been stored up over the years; the hurts, sadness, anger, resentment, and fear. He likens it to a negative energy field that we need to pay attention to.

> *"This accumulated pain is a negative energy field that occupies your body and mind. If you look on it as an invisible entity in its own right, you are getting quite close to the truth. It's the emotional pain-body. It has two modes of being: dormant and active. A pain-body may be dormant 90 percent of the time; in a deeply unhappy person, though, it may be active up to 100 percent of the time."—Eckhart Tolle.*

So, even if you think you are operating as an 'emotionally healthy person' in your daily life, your subconscious mind has recorded every little painful memory in its memory bank. It doesn't forget anything and these suppressed thoughts and memories live in you as stuck emotions that can manifest in eventual 'dis-ease.' Tolle suggests we become the watcher or witness of this pain body so that we can become separate from it. This technique is absolutely brilliant and helped me tremendously.

> *"So the pain-body doesn't want you to observe it directly and see it for what it is. The moment you observe it, feel its energy field within you, and take your attention into it, the identification is broken. A higher dimension of consciousness has come in. I call it presence. You are now the witness or the watcher of the pain-body. This means that it cannot use you anymore by pretending to be you, and it can no longer replenish itself through you. You have*

found your own innermost strength. You have accessed the power of now," Tolle states.

When you feel fear, anger, sadness or stuck in regret or unforgiveness, turn your attention to the pain and observe it. Observe it and then 'feel' the separateness of you the person, and the pain. Once you do this, you understand that you are not the pain and you are free.

Why did I get breast cancer at 37 years old? I really don't know for sure. But, I have my theories. One of those theories is the massive amount of stress I was under before it happened. Another theory is the unforgiveness in my heart towards my father.

I had unresolved emotions that I needed to expel that had been lingering for years and I needed to take a deeper look. I sensed that if I didn't do this work then I couldn't really move forward in the healthiest way possible. I wanted to be rid of any old emotional baggage that was holding me back from living an amazing, healthy life. And I wanted to be free of the fear.

What we know about disease is quite simple. Disease is caused by an imbalance in the body and energy field of the body. When we begin to heal our inner selves our immune system begins to self-regulate.

Stuck energy, or the pain body has also been coined as 'trapped emotions' by Dr. Bradley Nelson who does amazing work releasing emotions that cause physical issues within the body system.

Trapped emotions are the most common type of imbalance that human beings suffer from. They are invisible and can cause an amazing number of physical problems. They lower a person's immune function substantially and create an environment that is easy for disease to grow. They distort body tissue and block the flow of energy and disrupt the entire flow of the human healing system.

The process of becoming an observer of my pain-body helped me so much. It gave me a tool for my toolbox; an active way to stop the crazy emotions that were bombarding me. Every time I felt panicky and fearful, I would stop, become present and 'look' at my fear. Then I would acknowledge it. I would say out loud. "I see you fear!" I would feel better knowing that fear wasn't my natural state and I had the power to recognize it and separate from it.

"Pain can only feed on pain. Pain cannot feed on joy. It finds it quite indigestible." — *Eckhart Tolle*

Check in with yourself multiple times during the day. What are you feeling? How present are you? The more present you become with your difficult feelings, the more you can separate from them.

After my diagnosis, my intuition told me I had to move past the shock and the fear and start seeing a positive outcome for my illness. I had witnessed the pain and stayed in the scary place long enough. I was done. It was time to get to work and make a plan so I could live!

Chapter 4

Step 2

Get The Answers

"If you are unwell, don't ask to be healed, instead ask to be restored to that perfection from which you emanated." — Dr. Wayne Deyer.

Once I decided I had to shift my mindset, the right doctor appeared in my life. He knew exactly what to do to help me get well and it happened with ease. I let go of the constant fear and asked my higher power to reveal the right path for me. As soon as I relinquished the fear and struggle, that's when the right doctor for me came into my life.

My doctor was and is a very bright, positive light when I needed it most. I trusted him. I believed in him. I was overcome with happiness to find him. And this is the single most important thing to feel when you choose a doctor. There needs to be a rapport that is tangible. When I was in my doctor's presence, I felt uplifted and full of optimism and assurance that I would get completely well.

Many studies show that trust and rapport with your doctor plays an essential part in the healing process. Because of the peace I felt in surrendering my trust to him, I was able to focus on a different part of my healing process — the important things I could do on my own.

Doctors are conduits for healing. They don't actually heal you but are simply a vehicle for bringing about healing. If you don't connect with your doctor on some intrinsic level your subconscious mind won't trust the process and the connection may not be strong enough to allow you to heal in the best way possible.

Your belief system is so powerful that if you are convinced you have received real medicine instead of a placebo, your body will respond as if you have received the medicine and will heal. You must feel and believe that your doctor is a positive force in your healing process and has sincere intentions to help.

And beyond belief — you must have total faith in your practitioner. If you aren't comfortable you won't feel confident enough to talk to him or her about the most important and personal aspect of your life — your health! You have the right to know. You have the right to be involved. You have the right to question them until you are satisfied with all the answers. And I mean, all.

Another important thing to remember is, you can disagree, cry or even storm out of their office if you want to. Nobody is holding you hostage. Doctors can be intimidating and seem like they know everything, but they are not God and they don't have all the answers. They are human. We need them. We also need to ask them questions, check in with our intuition and maybe get two or three other opinions.

The first questions to consider asking:

Where is the cancer located exactly and what stage is it? You need to know specifics so you can be informed and can process what you're up against.

Can you recommend any colleagues to get a second opinion? When dealing with a life-threatening disease, it is an act of self-love and respect to get more than one opinion.

Which treatment do you recommend and why? It's important to know specifics because when you get another opinion, the answers may be different. You need to get all the advice possible so you can make an informed decision.

What is the goal for the treatment you are recommending? Usually the goal is to remove as much cancer as possible and find a way to make sure it doesn't come back. Your doctor's answer should satisfy you completely, then you can take the information and ask other physicians.

In your opinion, what are the chances of survival based on the treatment you are recommending? The answer you get here will be based on the standard western medical protocol for cancer. If you interview alternative physicians as well, you may get a different answer. All the information is helpful when deciding what course of action to take.

Getting a second or third opinion is important. Consulting with alternative physicians can also give you more information that you hadn't previously considered. You may come back to the same doctor after you've checked around.

Next — do the research and get some answers for yourself. Find out what you're up against. Read about the type of cancer you have and the various types of therapy offered, traditional and alternative. When I had breast cancer, I read lots of books and discovered a lot of important information that helped me. I also read a few wonderful books written by women who chose alternative paths and came out better than before cancer.

After the research, find a doctor that aligns with your thinking, someone you trust and have a rapport with before you begin your partnership in healing. I say partnership because that's what it is. You carry just as much responsibility in your healing process as the doctor does, if not more!

Being extraverted or feisty is welcome. Do not acquiesce to whatever the first thing your doctor tells you to do. Think about it. Feel your body. Does it feel right for you? Take a day, maybe two. Nothing bad will happen if you take a moment to feel and intuit. Trust yourself.

Did you know that statistically women who take an assertive approach in their healing process have a much better chance of survival?

How to Respectfully Disagree with Your Doctor

1. Be assertive in your approach.
2. Express your concerns honestly and ask your questions about the diagnosis or treatment.
3. Share why you disagree or what your concerns are.

4. Ask the doctor to explain their reasoning and provide more information.
5. Think of your healthcare as a partnership.

My doctor was very instrumental in keeping me hopeful and calm. He was so 'over-the-top' positive and happy every time I saw him that it super-sized the work I was doing to keep myself chugging along positively. He knew his stuff and I trusted him. He expected perfect results. So, why wouldn't I?

He wasn't giving me doom and gloom reports and telling me maybes and that I might die. He was literally singing Neil Diamond songs in the exam rooms with a smile. He knew that as a doctor that whatever he believed, I would most likely believe too. He knew that if he had a good attitude and emitted positive energy towards my healing process that I would be more positive and recover quicker. He understood the law of attraction for healing and how important it is to stay in a positive state in order to heal completely. I will forever be thankful to him for helping me heal.

Do you have rapport with your doctor? Does he or she make you feel like you can overcome the potential obstacles you are up against? If not, find someone else.

Chapter 5

Step 3

Become A Deliberate Thinker

"The soul always knows what to do to heal itself. The challenge is to silence the mind." — Caroline Myss

There's a crazy woman inside my head. Who is she? I've never met her before. Sound familiar? When we get cancer, we go a bit crazy at first. We don't recognize ourselves. In fact, we feel like we're living outside of our bodies. Time stops. It is a very strange phenomenon. Suddenly, we don't know anything. We are literally in shock and our thoughts go crazy. We feel we have no control over them — at all.

Most days it felt like I had an evil creature sitting on one shoulder and a beautiful angel on the other. One was telling me one thing and the other one quickly telling me the opposite. It went something like this:

I'm going to die and leave my baby motherless and then my husband is going to re-marry some horrible woman who won't know how to take care of our baby and the baby won't

like her because she's grieving the loss of her mother and my husband won't know how to handle it so they will fight a lot and that won't be good for the baby...

And then...

Stop it! you're going to be fine. This is not terminal and you can easily get through this with good positive energy and the right food and nutrition and with the amazing doctor you found and your higher power...

There are many versions of 'discussion' that go on in your head and if you have ever had cancer or any other life-threatening disease, you know this. It's a battle of the fittest and the mean, scary bully voice that thinks it knows everything is often the winner unless you sharpen your skills and learn how to beat it back into submission.

The goal is to step out of this network of thought chaos and work towards gaining control and becoming deliberate thinkers. Doesn't this sound empowering? We need to view our thoughts as tools to use to help elevate our vibratory frequency to a higher healing state and then micromanage them as best we can so they stay on course. They need to become our slaves and not vice versa.

I have spent years studying the power of the subconscious mind and the law of attraction. I know that whatever thoughts a person entertains the most are the ones that will attract equal results. And so here I was in a position now to really utilize, on a big scale, all the years of study I had put into the topic. But, could I do it? I had to. I felt that my life depended on it.

But, because a cancer diagnosis is usually a shock, it feels like there is no stopping the automatic negative thoughts that bombard us. All day long I was at war in my head and it was exhausting. Why couldn't I just be positive and be done with it? I had the tools. I had the knowledge. I was the perfect candidate for success.

Even with all my knowledge on the benefits of thinking positively, I realized I didn't have enough tools in my tool kit to handle this sort of life experience. If I was going to be successful I had to figure out a system to get my 'you're going to die and leave your child motherless' thoughts under control.

When we think of our thoughts we think of them generally in esoteric terms. But, did you know, thoughts are actually things? They are tangible, electrical frequencies. Did you know that thoughts can be measured?

Everything in the universe is made up of energy vibrating at different frequencies. Energy can neither be created nor can it be destroyed. Energy can only be transformed from one form to another. Your thoughts and feelings, including everything in your subconscious, are transmitting a particular vibration out into the universe, and those vibrations shape the life you are living.

However, as humans we forget how much power we have inside ourselves to initiate healing with our thoughts. We are the living, breathing embodiment of source energy. We have the same DNA as the stars and planets and all matter in the universe.

Dr. Joe Dispenza says it well when speaking on healing himself completely of a broken back.

> "First, every day I would put all of my conscious attention on this intelligence within me and give it a plan, a template, a vision, with very specific orders, and then I would surrender my healing to this greater mind that has unlimited power, allowing it to do the healing for me.

And second, I wouldn't let any thought slip by my awareness that I didn't want to experience."

I love that Dr. Dispenza wouldn't allow any thought to slip by that he didn't want to experience. When faced with a crisis, unless you have a well-trained mind and know how to handle your thoughts, they will most likely take you over and 'become you.' It is important to become a micromanager of your thoughts.

Ten percent of our brains are our conscious minds and the other 90% is our subconscious mind. The subconscious is like a secret inner stenographer, recording our lives, that never lies and never cheats. Whatever you instruct it to do, it will do. The subconscious has the power to cure illness in your body and your mind. It knows how to heal you if you tell it to.

If you are thinking about, talking about or imagining about your disease, you need to be careful because you are attracting the illness frequency that you are trying to get rid of.

The subconscious mind has a large part in determining your health. It knows how you really feel. It knows your pain, your anger, your entire life, second by second. It knows everything that has ever happened to you. If your thoughts are negative, your body will reflect that in the way you feel.

There is an emerging field of science called psychoneuroimmunology that demonstrates the connection between the mind and the body.

"Your every thought produces a biochemical reaction in the brain. The brain then releases chemical signals that are transmitted to the body, where they act as the messen-

gers of the thought. The thoughts that produce the chemicals in the brain allow your body to feel exactly the way you were just thinking." — Dr. Joe Dispenza

The connection between your mind and your body could be compared to a switchboard that is working in unison. The subconscious can help you heal your illness by connecting with your higher self — The 'conscious you' or 'the greater mind' or whatever you wish to call it, that is now paying attention.

We can't *not* think about our diagnoses. But, we can choose what thoughts we think to a large degree. Many thoughts are automatic. Experts estimate that the mind thinks between 60,000 to 80,000 thoughts per day. That's an average of 2,500 to 3,300 thoughts per hour. Research has proved that all thought carries a vibrational frequency.

Revered philosopher, Ralph Waldo Emerson said,

"We become what we think about all day long."

We are not victims to our thoughts. We are the boss of them. Don't let them run wild like stallions. Tame them! Become a deliberate thinker.

When you think healthy thoughts it's also crucial that you feel good when doing it. Nothing will change if you say rote affirmations. You have to feel it and believe that you are getting well! You have to muster up all the faith inside your being to feel that not only are you getting well, but that you are thriving! Meditation allows for this process. Even if you only commit to 10 to 20 minutes a day to sit and be still and breathe and imagine yourself perfectly well and really feel it, this will help tremendously or see my guided meditations for more help to get to the quantum field space of healing. Miracles happen in this space.

If you can't get any positive emotions mustered up, think about your child or your dog or something you truly love and feel the love in your heart. Then, while you are in that state, take the love feeling and shift it over to your thoughts of being perfectly healthy. Feel the loving emotions as you image yourself completely well. Even for just a few seconds throughout your day — stop and close your eyes, see yourself completely well and really feel the gratefulness in your heart. Feel it as deeply as you can! It only takes a few seconds. I did this multiple times throughout the day. Every positive emotion you feel adds up to the greater good for healing. In the morning and night you can do longer versions.

"I no longer create by default. I am a deliberate thinker. I think on purpose. I speak on purpose. I act on purpose."
— Abraham Hicks

During my bout with breast cancer I realized I had to slow things down and take a look at my thoughts. But, how on earth do you manage your thoughts? We have so many of them. Thousands every day!

I didn't really know what to do at first, so I just started paying attention. I practiced mindfulness and observed the thoughts when they came into my mind. In fact, I would say I started to police my thoughts like a general in the army. I observed the dramatic, scary, often death thoughts as they entered my mind and, before the emotion could grab and control me, I would visualize the thought in a circle and strike it out with a line (like a 'no dogs' sign) and say, sometimes out loud —

I CANCEL THAT THOUGHT!

With conviction.

If the thought came back, which often it did, I would repeat the process. Then I would replace the thought with a positive one. For instance,

"I am getting healthier every day!" or "My body heals perfectly!"

In the beginning, this process would go on throughout my day and I would be cancelling thoughts left and right! After a while, the scary thoughts became less and less frequent. I would still get some negative thoughts creeping in occasionally, but now I knew what to do to switch them off.

I noticed something else; observing the thoughts took away their power immediately.

Nobody can control all of their thoughts all the time and I certainly couldn't control all of mine when I was dealing with breast cancer. I did the best I could, but there were plenty of times that I would struggle with it. In those moments I chose to forgive myself, sit quietly and just observe the negativity, bear witness to it and then allow it to drift away. Like a toddler having a tantrum, I would allow the thoughts to go crazy and then I would say, sometimes out loud. "Okay, that's enough! Good bye crazy thoughts!" or "Thank you, moving on now!" etc. And then I would replace the thoughts with the positive ones.

The process of training our mind is not that different from an athlete training for the Olympics. When something big is happening in our lives, (figure skating in the Olympics or dealing with cancer) we need to pay very close attention to our training. We also need to understand that when we fail, which we will, we just dust ourselves off and get back to what we have learned in our training. The training techniques work and we know we can rely on them. When we fall or slip up, we get back on our feet and try again.

Everything changed when I changed my mindset. The fear that was paralyzing me no longer had a grip. My thoughts were now tools for me to manipulate to my advantage. I started using them as fuel for healing. Whenever a negative thought arose, I would cancel it and replace it with an emotionally charged, happy and healing thought about my body. I was becoming a deliberate thinker.

Chapter 6

Step 4

WATCH YOUR WORDS — YOUR MIND IS LISTENING

"A single word has the power to influence the expression of genes that regulate physical and emotional stress." — Dr. Andrew Newberg, Dr. Mark Robert Waldman from the book 'Words Can Change Your Brain.'

Sticks and stones can break my bones, but words will never hurt me? **Wrong.**

Dr. Newberg and Dr. Waldman state that positive words strengthen the frontal lobe in our brains and the more we concentrate on them the more we are benefited, whereas negatively charged words have the opposite effect. A single negatively charged word can increase the activity in our amygdala (the fear center of the brain), releasing a mass of stress hormones and neurotransmitters.

Words have power. We don't consider this fact much. When we speak, the words mostly just roll out of our mouths without much thought. Some of us are more conscious when we speak and try to choose our words more wisely, but not to the degree we should.

The word 'cancer' has a negative charge to it. In the 1950's specific advertising campaigns were created to engrain the fear of cancer in the general population. Later, 'Cancer phobia' created by the fear campaigns was coined in an article by Dr. George Crile, Jr., in Life Magazine, in 1955. His insight describe conditions today as accurately as they did then.

> *"Those responsible for telling the public about cancer have chosen the weapon of fear, believing that only through fear can the public be educated. Newspapers and magazines have magnified and spread this fear, knowing that the public is always interested in the melodramatic and the frightening. This has fostered a disease, fear of cancer, a contagious disease that spreads from mouth to ear. It is possible that today, in terms of the total number of people affected, fear of cancer is causing more suffering than cancer itself. This fear leads both doctors and patients to do unreasonable and therefore dangerous things."*

You may be thinking, can words really affect our healing? Well, we know that all things in the universe are made of energy, whether they breathe or not. The beginning of creation was sound and every sound carries a vibrational frequency. Words when spoken carry a vibrational frequency just as a thought does and therefor words have the power to affect and influence us based on that vibration.

Words such as love, joy, peace and happy carry positive vibrations. Words like hate, anger and sad have a negative frequency. Similarly, the vibrational frequency of the word 'cancer' is negative.

Japanese scientist, Masaru Emoto, who wrote, 'The Hidden Messages of Water,' performed some amazing experiments in the 1990s on the effect that words have on energy. In his experiments, Emoto poured water into laboratory vials that were labeled with negative words like "I hate you" or "fear." After 24 hours the water produced gray, misshapen clumps instead of beautiful lace-like crystals. In contrast, Emoto placed labels that said things like "I Love You," or "Peace" on vials of polluted water, and after 24 hours, they produced gleaming, perfectly hexagonal crystals. Emoto's experiments proved that energy generated by positive or negative words can actually change the physical structure of an object.

Every time you say the word 'cancer' you are giving it attention and affirming it. Every time you say, "I have breast cancer" you affirm the disease in your body and reinforce its presence. Think about that for a moment.

I rarely talked about breast cancer when I had it or afterwards. When I was out with friends or family, I would talk about other things. I didn't want to linger in the vibration of fear and disease any more than I was already and I understood that the more attention I put on it, the more power I was giving it.

I also thought that if I told people I had breast cancer they would look at me differently. Their concern for me would translate into a vibration of worry and fear and I didn't want that energy around me. I wanted to be treated as if I was normal and healthy. I didn't want to ruminate on the negative.

I stopped using the word cancer and I stopped telling people I had it. Once I had the surgery to remove the tumor, I spoke and behaved as if I was completely healthy. I had cancer in my body and then I didn't anymore. It was gone. If it's gone — why talk about it? I felt no need.

The more we talk about our illness, the more we perpetuate it. The negative frequency grows and grows like a vortex of bad energy around us. Don't ruminate endlessly and discuss your situation over and over with your friends, family or strangers that you meet. Let it be. Don't pick the scab and make it worse.

Breast cancer is <u>not</u> a part of who you are. It's a temporary condition. Cancer cells are merely cells that have gone rogue. Everyone has rogue cancer cells in their bodies, just some people's immune systems aren't able to fight them off for a variety of reasons. When we understand this, the story isn't as scary anymore. Remember, you are a healthy person with a temporary condition and that condition is in the process of being eliminated from your body.

Cancer is a heavy word — like cement. Nobody thinks positively when they hear that word. The more we talk about illness, the more we cement it into our subconscious mind. We need to concentrate on balancing our bodily system. All illnesses are just symptoms of physical imbalance and emotional baggage. No illness can remain when the entire physical and emotional system is in balance!

We also need to change the way we create dialogue around cancer. We hear these phrases a lot; *diagnosed with cancer, cancer victim, cancer patient, battling cancer, cancer survivor.* These every day phrases are the language of cancer, ingrained in our discourse. The way we talk about a disease we're facing can affect how we feel about it, and those feelings can impact us and our ability to heal faster.

How do these words make you feel? They make me feel heavy, sad and scared.

Choosing our words carefully can change our feelings about an illness. Some ideas include, instead of "I have cancer", you could say *"I was diagnosed with"*...Think about it — the doctors aren't diagnosing YOU, the human being, they are diagnosing the disease.

Danielle Ofri, MD, PhD, an internist at New York University School of Medicine points out: "I'd rather say that a person 'had cancer' and leave it in the past tense." Dr. Dizon continues: "Cancer is a noun, not an adjective."

It's healthy to talk about our fears and struggles, no doubt. We need to express all of our fears and concerns. However, it is best not to go on and on about our cancer diagnosis. It is best not to keep ruminating on it and reading about it and talking about it. I'm not saying be in denial, not at all. You already know you have or had cancer, so there is no reason to keep discussing it with friends and family, obsessing over it. Choose the words around your illness carefully and use them sparingly.

Then there's the word; survivor. You hear a lot of women who have had breast cancer say, *"I'm a survivor."* They wear it like a badge of honor. But, cancer is not a part of your natural personal identity so why are you so proud?

I say — let it go!

Just being alive makes us survivors. People survive wars and all sorts of tragedies. Life has its challenges. How do we measure the weight of a challenge?

How we talk about having cancer should be a choice. I don't want to be labelled as a survivor just because it's 'the thing to do.' To me, the word survivor is a sad word. It has the vibratory frequency of victimhood and I don't want people to feel sorry for me because I endured something difficult.

Other diseases don't create survivors after the person is healed. No one says that they are a malaria survivor, or an aneurism survivor, even though these diseases can be quite deadly. Even doctors agree that not all patients after cancer identify as survivors, so we should not assume it is an all-embraced term.

How about, "I'm dealing with a cancer issue" or "I had to deal with a cancer issue but I'm well now." These sorts of words and statements avoid burying our personal identity in a disease.

The word survivor creates a badge of sorts. It singles you out as special. It can give you attention and part of you may like that but this kind of attention is not in your best interest. The word survivor infers a great struggle and that we almost didn't make it. Okay sure, that may have happened but why do we need to announce it? Why is it so important to hang on to the story of pain and suffering and let everyone know about it? It's just one story in a life time of stories!

Ask yourself — are you using this title as a scapegoat to allow yourself to feel sorry for yourself? Do you like it when people treat you differently than if you didn't have breast cancer? Does what I'm saying make you feel upset because you may have to let go of a title that you feel you earned by struggling? If anything, survivorship should be a temporary state of being and then released when you are free of cancer. Why hold on to it? Be free!

After I had my surgery and I was on my healing path, I had to get back to my life. One day I heard about a walk for breast cancer in Malibu where I was living. Cindy Crawford was sponsoring it and I thought...*huh, maybe that's something I should do. I can get out there with Cindy and walk a few miles in support of breast cancer. Why not?*

So on the day of the walk, I showed up at the event and noticed two separate registration points for sign up purposes. The first had a big sign that said, 'Survivors' and the second sign had a sign that said, 'Guest.'

While I watched everyone march up to each of the posts without any consideration, I found myself frozen. I didn't know which one of these labels fit me best. I didn't feel like a survivor at all. I felt like I had conquered something, but not survived it.

I felt more like a guest but for some reason I went to the survivor line because that is what I thought society's expectations would have me do. I had the volunteer stick a survivor sign on my front and back. Afterwards, she smiled at me but I could tell she felt sorry for me. I could feel her thought process bury right into my soul. *Who is this young, pretty woman? What happened to her? Oh, how sad.* I hated the feeling I was getting from her. It made me feel singled out and weak. I wanted to tell her that I was fine and I would be fine and not to worry about me.

As I walked in the woods, I noticed a lot of people looking at my sign. They would look at the sign, then at me and then their thought bubbles would appear.

Poor girl. How sad. She's so young.

I noticed Cindy Crawford looking at me with the same curious look. I started to get very uncomfortable because I felt like a fraud. I wasn't a survivor. I was happy. I was grateful to be alive and grateful for the experience because it had put me on an incredible healing journey. I was living my best life now. It took wearing a sign on my back to realize I was not a survivor, nor did I ever want to be.

When I got home I stood in front of my husband and showed him my sign. He looked at me curiously, kind of confused. I asked him what he thought. Did he think of me as a survivor? He thought about it and then casually said he didn't and then asked me why I was wearing it. I told him that I didn't know.

I tossed the sign off my back and felt a huge sense of relief. Then I threw it in the trash. Goodbye sad word! Now, if they had a sign that said, 'conqueror,' I would have worn that sign with pleasure. Because words have power and I was not a survivor or a victim. I was a victor, a conqueror.

These words may seem meaningless however they carry great weight whether we realize it or not. What we label ourselves in our lives matters. Words have power, especially when you literally stick them on your body and claim to be what the words say.

When you identify with words, choose positive, life-affirming, powerful words. I am healthy! I am powerful! I am a conquerer! I overcome any obstacle!

Remission is another word that I never use. The true story is; I had the surgery to remove the lump in my breast and now it is gone. After surgery, there was no trace in my body of cancer, therefore the cancer is gone. Remission infers very strongly that it is sort of hanging around and could pounce back like a wild tiger at any moment.

Even if you have some cancer remaining in your body, why do you want to be reminded of that by labelling yourself that way? Wouldn't it be more productive to say that you are getting healthier every day? Why must the medical establishment insist that we go into a state of remission? What purpose does it really serve? It keeps us in trepidation, that some day the cancer might come back. It keeps us in fear.

Here is the definition of remission:

Remission: a temporary or permanent decrease or subsidence of manifestations of a disease, a period during which such a decrease or subsidence occurs.

A temporary decrease for a period of time? That is not how I choose to word my healed body. Why would anyone want to? If I labelled myself in remission I would be walking around every day wondering when the cancer was coming back. It is a power sucking word that makes you, once again, the victim of circumstance. Being in a 'maybe it will come back one day' state of mind is not healthy and subconsciously allows your mind to stay in a state of preparation just in case. No thanks!

Once we understand the damage these words can do to our health, we need to stop using them and replace them with other words. Instead of using the word cancer consistently, try focusing on healthy and happier words such as, recovery, improving, thriving, conquering. We had an illness but we're better now. Replacing fear-based words with high frequency words has a physiological effect on our bodies. There is evidence to show that positive words heal us.

So shift your words, stop talking about disease and get well!

Chapter 7

Step 5

Reclaim Your Power

Throughout history women have often put themselves second. We tend to put our husbands, boyfriends, partners, children and sometimes even our friends first. Why? Because we are by nature caring and nurturing and we often forget to nurture ourselves.

Sometimes women put themselves on the road to illness because they aren't living their authentic lives and then when they get an illness they go into victim mode and agree to whatever their doctors tell them to do.

Many women acquiesce to men, family, friends and children and feel the need to be nice or polite to others instead of expressing their true feelings. We often don't believe in ourselves. To top it off sometimes we blame our significant other in our lives for our problems. By placing the blame on our partner we don't need to look at ourselves. This isn't something new.

The word victim infers weakness. We don't want to be victims in life. We want to be strong and deliberate creators in life. Living in victimhood where we don't feel in control of our own destiny can contribute to a sense of powerlessness. Women who don't live in their power can't own their truth and can't express themselves in an authentic way. They suppress emotions and live in physical discord separate from their soul nature, which is peace.

Dr. Ernest H. Rosenbaum from Stanford University Medical Center brilliantly states:

> *"The best thing a patient can do to strengthen the will to live is to get involved as an active participant in combating his or her disease. When patients approach their disease in an aggressive fighting posture, they are no longer helpless victims. Instead, they become active partners with their medical support team in the fight for improvement or cure. This partnership must be based on honesty, open communication, shared responsibility, and education about the nature of the disease, therapy options, and rehabilitation. The result of this partnership is an increased ability to cope that, in turn, nurtures the will to live.*
>
> *As you make the transition from helpless victim to activist, one of the most important realizations is that you have everything to do with how others perceive you and treat you. If you can accept your condition and hold self-pity at bay, others won't feel sorry for you. If you can discuss your disease and medical therapy in a matter-of-fact manner, they'll respond in kind without fear or awkwardness. You are in charge. You can subtly and gently put your family, friends, and coworkers at ease by being frank about what you want to talk about or not talk about and by being explicit about whether and when you want their help."*

When we begin to embrace ourselves just as we are and

live authentically, we release mental and physical friction from our lives. Do you know who you really are? If not, I will tell you: *You are a spiritual being having a human experience.* As a spiritual being you have more power than you will ever know!

You have the ability to heal yourself. You have the ability to manifest beautiful experiences in your life. But, sometimes we forget who we are. We are not living our authentic lives. We have forgotten the power we have and don't know how to tap into it.

We need to find peace within ourselves. Find the joy of who we are right now. We need to release our shame, guilt, sadness, anger and dissatisfactions. But, how do we do that? I believe the moment we accept ourselves just as we are, right now, we start the process of full healing.

Are you happy with who you are? Do you accept yourself just as you are, faults and imperfections included? Accepting and loving ourselves can be difficult, but we have to get there. We have to forgive ourselves for not being the person we think we should be. Right here, right now, you can accept yourself just the way you are. You don't need to be any different from who you are in this moment. You are perfect just as you are. Say it out loud...

I am enough. Just the way I am.

We are all just human beings trying to figure it out. We all have faults. We have done some questionable things in our lives, we have been lied to and perhaps lied to others, we have been abandoned, abused or not taken seriously, and most of us have not lived up to our true potential. That's because this life is a journey and we will forever be striving and seeking because our potential is limitless. So, then when is the perfect time to start accepting ourselves? We will never be perfect. Things will never be perfect. Life is messy. So, wouldn't now be a good time?

Every morning, say, "I am enough" in the mirror, with feeling. It only takes a second or two. Things will shift very quickly for you. And when you stumble and feel annoyed or dissatisfied with yourself, say it again. I am enough. Repeat until you feel good. Write it on your mirror, put notes on your fridge, put it as a screensaver on your phone. Do whatever it takes to remind yourself that you are enough, just as you are. I highly recommend the wisdom of Dr. Marisa Peer in the area of claiming the simple, yet powerful philosophy of 'I am enough' to transform your life. You can find her work online.

To live authentically is to know and accept ourselves just as we are, right now. Being authentic is about getting to the core of your way of being and forgiving yourself for not being perfect. Living authentically takes courage but what is this life for if we can't be our true selves and express to the world the gifts that we have been given? Do we need everyone's approval in life? No, we don't.

Once you make the choice to follow authentic living, here are some ways to start to connect with your authentic self and embrace it in your whole being:

Start with becoming aware of how you're truly feeling, be with those emotions, and practice communicating this to yourself and others. This will help your body to feel safe in the face of authenticity. Practicing mindfulness through meditation can also help you become the watcher of your feelings and sensations in your body, helping you to become more in tune with your inner experience.

Take deep breaths, into your stomach, often throughout the day. Believe it or not, the simplest tool to connect us with the core of who we are is our breath. This is why many ancient traditions have relied upon breath work to connect with our authentic self. Try the ancient method of the 4-7-8 breathing that we covered earlier.

Become aware of your learned tendencies, or parts of you that feel the need to jump into action to help live a life for others. This could include: people pleasing, being a caretaker, taskmaster, over achiever, distractor, or worrier. We all have these sub-personality parts of ourselves that make us feel accepted. These parts of ourselves usually resist change when we decide to move into a more authentic way of being.

Calming your nervous system. Many of us who have strong tendencies to be who others want us to be do so because of traumatic experiences we've had in our lives. To start feeling safe around being our authentic self, we can stop and listen to what our inner voice tells us that we need. We can practice mindfulness by being more present — observing our thoughts and actions and living more from a place of ease and calm instead of fight or flight.

Women who have had breast cancer are often dealing with long standing emotional pain, usually anger and unforgiveness. Sometimes, we don't even realize we are carrying this heavy weight around. But our bodies do!

Loren Toussaint, a psychologist at Luther College who has worked as a consultant and has written a book on health and forgiveness, says there is evidence that cancer patients who report poor quality of life don't do as well. He thinks emotional well-being deserves more attention.

Toussaint said: "Forgiveness, I think, has its largest role

to play in helping people to cope with the psychosocial fallout of cancer." He said there's strong evidence that stress leaves people worn down mentally and physically. Being angry at others, he said, activates the same kinds of physiological responses as other kinds of stress.

There are seven chakras starting from the base of the spine and ending at the top of the head. Each chakra supplies life energy to its surrounding organs. If one of them is out of alignment, the whole body suffers. The breast area represents the fourth or heart chakra. The heart chakra is associated with love, forgiveness and compassion — qualities of the heart. Breast cancer is caused by a disturbance in the energy flow in this chakra.

When I was about ten years old, my dad left the family. I remember peering out the living room window as he drove away with a mattress on top of his car. He never came back and never paid any money to take care of his three daughters. In fact, he fought my mother in court so he wouldn't have to pay for us.

I don't remember feeling particularly sad, mostly just anxious. I must have internalized my feelings because when it came time to do 'the work' with a therapist, I discovered a great deal of hurt, anger and unforgiveness towards my father that I hadn't really been aware of. It was an incredible revelation for me.

I realized I needed to work through the hurt and anger and forgive him. At my therapist's instruction, I wrote a letter to my father and expressed all of my feelings. I'll never forget the pain and anger that flowed from my pen once I started to release my feelings on the page. It was truly cathartic. And I didn't think I had any issues with my dad! But, the subconscious knows all and that exercise allowed me to expel the pain that I had stored up since I was a child. After I wrote the letter, I was instructed to burn it.

It was a simple but powerful act. I understood that by forgiving my father, I was healing myself. It was a very transformative time in my life. Dis-ease creates disease. I realized my body was storing my hurt, anger, sadness and pain in various parts of my body. And when I learned how to release them, I felt liberated. I worked through the issue and came out the other side, softer and more relaxed. The experience was empowering.

In order to reclaim our power, we need to release old stuck emotions from our bodies. This may include pain from:

- Any traumatic event / PTSD
- Home life, work situations
- Chronic stress
- Physical injury or illness
- Abuse
- Internalizing your feelings
- Divorce or relationship problems
- Rejection, betrayal, or abandonment
- Loss of a loved one
- Negative self-talk
- Negative beliefs about oneself or others (e.g., "I am not good enough" or "I do not deserve to heal / receive love / etc.")
- Unforgiveness; hatred towards others

Every emotion has its own energetic frequency. In his book Power vs. Force, Dr. David Hawkins discusses the "Map of Consciousness" — a scale showing the energetic frequencies of specific emotions, with negative emotions calibrating at much lower frequencies than positive ones.

Because we are all energetic beings, these emotional energies affect us down to the atomic level and have an impact on our health and our lives. Clearing them away removes all sorts of roadblocks to healing ourselves, in a similar way that acupuncture strengthens the life force of the body.

Reflections

- Do you consider yourself a caring, nurturing person, prone to being over-caring?
- Do you mostly put your needs last?
- What resentment do you need to let go of? Whom do you need to forgive?
- What emotional memories do you still need to heal? Are there any relationships in your life that require healing?
- Who are the people that you are yet to forgive and what prevents you from letting go of the pain associated with them?
- Do you ever use emotional wounds to control people or situations?
- What have you done that needs forgiving? Which people are working to forgive you?

We need to understand and acknowledge that it is our divine birthright to be healthy. We don't need to give away our power to others by living in a place of unforgiveness or anger at what life has dealt us. Surrender the old hurts and pain that others have inflicted upon you. It is not your burden to carry. It never was. We make life what we want it to be. We are deliberate creators capable of great health and happiness. And we can choose that right now.

Yesterday is just an old story and tomorrow doesn't even exist. There is only right now and in the now you can choose to be the powerful being that you were born to be. Choose that person every day and watch your life transform!

Chapter 8

Step 6

Get To The Happy Place

Breast cancer isn't fun and it doesn't offer much to smile about. It definitely doesn't make us happy. So, how on earth do we get to the happy place when we have breast cancer? Is it even possible? I believe it is. It takes work to get out of the fearful place, but it is possible. I know, because I did it!

We can't escape suffering and suddenly be happy. We need to seek resources that allow us to engage in the suffering safely — observe it, express and release it in a healthy way with therapy, writing in a journal or writing a letter to the person who hurt us (and then burn it) or other constructive ways.

After I went through my fear and panic stage during my bout with breast cancer, I made it a goal to get to a place where I felt positive and happy, at least for most of the time. All of the techniques I have shared in this book helped me to get there. I didn't do it in a day. But, I did make it a priority. Some people truly thought I was in denial because I was pretty happy all the time. I could hear the thought bubbles...

Why is she smiling? Why does she seem happy? Doesn't she have breast cancer?

Just because we have or had breast cancer doesn't mean we need to act 'appropriately' by being sad and scared!

Just by going through breast cancer, you are already in the process of overcoming and building resiliency and therefore, happiness. In fact, you have been overcoming your entire life. Think about it. Challenges at school, with friends, with family members, with work. You have overcome challenges and built a foundation of success just based on your life. It's how you process it, accept it, forgive others and yourself and then move on that counts.

I used many tools to get me to the happy place during my bout with breast cancer. One of them was walking in nature, specifically in forests. There is evidence growing worldwide that spending at least 20 minutes in green spaces provides an increase in wellbeing, happiness and improves overall mental and physical health. In 2018, NHS Shetland, a government-run hospital system in Scotland, began allowing doctors at ten medical establishments to write nature prescriptions for their patients as a routine part of patient care. Dr. Chloe Evans at Scalloway Health centre states: "I want to take part because the project provides a structured way for patients to access nature as part of a non-drug approach to health problems."

Nature heals our minds, bodies and souls. It makes us happy. Get out of the house and find your nearest park and walk for 20 minutes and 'forest bathe'. Immerse yourself in the nature and forget about your problems. Move your body, breathe the air, appreciate the nature and be present.

Doing the work; eating well, taking inventory of our past, seeking the right course of healing for ourselves, micromanaging our thoughts and words, and actively seeking solutions for our health is a road map for happiness. The act of taking responsibility for our lives and making it better is the first step. You don't have to be at the end of the journey to feel the happiness. You can be in the beginning or the middle and just knowing that you have a plan that feels good, that you are being pro-active, doing the work on your own behalf — this is positive and affirming and this brings about the happiness.

Sometimes we need quick fixes. We need to feel good right now because we are once again spiralling into fear. If you google how to get happy quick — it will tell you seven ways to do this that take less than a minute. Some of these ways include counting our blessings, thinking of a loved one, saying a quick affirmation or doing a 45 second meditation. I know when I sit still for a few moments and think about my loved ones and give thanks for them, my heart swells with love and happiness. Keeping the vibration up and humming is key. Even though we can't just snap our fingers and be happy, we can use these tools to get us out of the panic place that we can easily slip into when faced with disease.

The 51 percent rule suggests if we keep our thoughts positive over 50 percent, we will have tipped the balance to success. That may seem like an impossible task when dealing with a life-threatening disease. You may be thinking you're only at five or ten percent. That's okay. Changing our mind-set happens bit by bit. It takes presence and determination. Be patient with yourself and just keep repeating the steps over and over until your mind finally gets the 'aha' moment and does what you ask it to do. Getting over the 50 percent mark requires paying close attention to how we're feeling. Being the watcher of our thoughts and practicing daily meditation brings the feeling of positivity and happiness into our lives.

Research shows that laughter and happiness have a direct effect on our immune system. Steve Cole, a psychoneuroimmunologist who studies the link between mind and body healing did a study and found that participants that had a purpose-based outlook had significant gene-expression profiles effecting their immune systems in a positive way. People that find their way out of victimhood and get involved with a purpose, thrive.

This study and others like it prove that happiness based on living a purposeful life affects our immune system in ways we have no idea about. It also takes our minds off our problems when we focus on something other than ourselves or someone else's issues. When we are helping others, or involved in a creative or intellectual pursuit, our energetic field lights up with excitement and happiness and we naturally heal our mind and body simultaneously without even knowing it.

You may be wondering how on earth you can start thinking about helping others when you need to help yourself. Shouldn't we be completely focused on our health? It's a good question. And the answer is yes and no. Yes, you need to hyper focus on many things to get yourself well, but we are amazing human beings capable of doing many things at once and focusing on someone else's needs not only helps another human being, but also releases the feel-good hormones that contribute to our healing. Is there someone in your neighbourhood that needs help? Is there a charity you can volunteer at? Is there a friend who could use a ride to buy groceries? The best way to stop ruminating on our health issues is to help someone else.

If we're not careful, breast cancer likes to make victims

out of us. Sometimes women have a hard time finding their way out of this space. Sometimes, they don't even know they are in it. Perhaps their mother was also a victim in life and it's a learned behaviour and feels natural. It's easy to get caught up in feeling sorry for ourselves. The trick is to become aware of how you are feeling in the present moment, more often.

Ask yourself right now — am I deliberately creating a positive future for my health by choosing to grow and learn and seek positivity and goodness in my life? Or, am I choosing to remain in a place of despair and sadness because it's easier and more comfortable?

Actively seeking positivity and happiness is a choice. It doesn't happen just by snapping our fingers — we need to really want it and understand that it helps us get through the fire to the other side in a healthier way, mentally and physically.

Accept yourself just as you are, love yourself, forgive yourself and those who have hurt you. You are enough just as you are! Find joy in your pursuits and learn to train your mind and emotions. Be the master of your thoughts and words. Understand that feelings aren't facts. You are the boss of your life and have more control than you realize. Become a deliberate thinker and creator. When you do this, every single day, your immune system will recalibrate and heal you.

Feel it. See it. Believe it. Know it.

Part Three

Nutrition For The Body, Mind & Soul

Chapter 9

The Happy Healing Project

When I was going through breast cancer, I named my healing process, 'The Happy Healing Project' because I wanted to have a positive reference point to go back to in those moments when I was slipping back into doubt and fear. The word 'happy' has power and a positive frequency and just thinking and saying the word made me feel positive about the path I had chosen for myself. The word 'healing' was exactly what I wanted for myself and the word 'project' gave me purpose. It made me feel focused and committed to the job that I had to do. Between all the negative chatter and energy around cancer, I needed that positive home-base to find my center whenever I felt bad. I also used other high frequency words to help me.

Studies show that if you read or say positive words out loud to yourself it increases wellbeing in your body. If you begin with 'I am' it is even more powerful. So I started reading a list of words and I couldn't really believe it but I immediately felt better. Just reading them lightened me. Here is some of the list:

Love, happiness, peace, blessed, success, comfort, laugh, nurture, support, understanding, peace, safe, healthy.

Or, I am loving, happy, blessed, successful, comforted, laughing, nurtured, supported, understood, peaceful, safe, healthy.

I practiced happiness daily. I meditated, I read affirming words. I created an 'I am' list. I read inspiration healing stories, which there are many. I watched funny movies. I walked in nature. I laughed with my daughter. I didn't talk about cancer. I avoided negative people and chatter. I avoided bad news on t.v. to keep my happiness frequency up. I protected it like a fragile child! I took my Happy Healing Project seriously.

Find things that make you happy and repeat them daily. Develop positive habits. Identify the things that make you unhappy, and work toward eliminating them from your life. Keep the negative or doubting people in your life at a distance. It's a project of separation, and when you master it, it's a helpful strategy for how to be happy. Self-healing requires commitment. Intentionally creating happiness during the process requires mindfulness.

As we all know there is no point in doing anything worthwhile, half-baked. The more important the thing we need to do is — the more we need to commit. I would say that staying healthy and alive may be the single most important thing a person could do. Wouldn't you?

You need to apply your will power. Remember, your mind controls the will and your will controls the energy. It is not the will that heals but the energy, stirred up by the will that effects a healing. There is no force more effective than energy applied through will power roused by a positive mind.

As the Indian Master, Paramahansa Yogananda said:

"Will and energy are the two most effective powers in the bodily system." Your will-power controls the healing energy in your body.

On a subatomic level, your body is just materialized energy and that energy can be controlled by will.

"Divine Will is omnipresent and is the sole creative and sustaining power in the universe, residing in every unit of cosmic energy... therefore to send sufficient energy into the body to bring about divine healing requires that you connect your will with the all-powerful creative will of God." — Paramahansa Yogananda.

All I had to do was look at my new baby to give me the strength and confidence I needed to get well. This supercharged my faith and my willpower. She made me so happy. I used the happiness I felt when I was with my baby and transmuted it into a healing energy for myself.

We are born perfect. Have faith that you can return to that perfect healthy state. Faith is knowing through intuitive perception which occurs when you are one with truth. Belief, on the other hand, can be changed by a contradictory opinion.

My words and this book will not help you heal if you have doubt. You have to shift your mind into a new paradigm of absolute knowing that you will be well. You have to know it so deeply that no matter what anyone says, your knowing stays intact. To get you to this state and to stay there more often, I have created a series of powerful guided meditations to help you. (See my website for details at holisticbreastexpert.com)

Faith and knowing is the best way to shift matter inside your body to bring about absolute healing!

Daily steps

1. In the morning, instead of laying in bed thinking about all the bad stuff — GET UP. Don't lay there and ruminate. The moment you wake up, force yourself to get your body out of the bed. The bed can be a dangerous place for falling back into old patterns and it's important to start your day off positive from the very beginning. Once you propel yourself out of bed, and before your feet touch the ground, say out loud or in your mind: THANK YOU FOR MY HEALING TODAY! I AM GETTING HEALTHIER AND HEALTHIER EVERY DAY! TODAY IS AN AMAZING DAY FULL OF LOVE AND MIRACLES FOR MY HEALTH! Say it with conviction.
2. When you get up and brush your teeth, etc., thank The Creator/The Universe/Source Energy, or whatever you like to call it, for at least five things you are grateful for and REALLY FEEL the love, joy and warmth surrounding it. It could be your child, your husband, your cat, your rose garden, etc. The energy and peace you will feel from this will supercharge your emotions and set you on the right track. You can then transfer those good feelings to thoughts of your health and affirm, Thank you for my healing today! I am healthy, whole and happy.
3. Meditate for at least 10 to 20 minutes (or longer!) morning and night. When you turn off external nervous energy and calm yourself in

meditation and your life-force takes a break from all your senses, you connect with your higher power. If you don't have a practice already, I recommend mindfulness meditation or go to Self-Realization Fellowship for instruction on their beautiful practice of meditation. The results of this simple practice will amaze you. (I am a certified meditation teacher in mindfulness meditation so if you want more information, please contact me at heidi@holisticbreastexpert.com.) Everything you do in your day should be done with peace and love in mind. Try to hold on to the feeling of peace and love within you after your meditation.

4. Commit to micro-managing your thoughts. Every time you see your thoughts turning to the negative (and they will) bring them back to center and replace them with a positive thought.

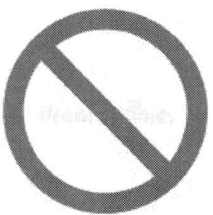

1. If the thought is really bad, close your eyes and in your mind put it in a red circle with a

diagonal line through it and say — I CANCEL THAT THOUGHT! And move on with your day. I did this hundreds of times during my recovery. It works!

2. Don't use phrases like, I HAVE CANCER or I AM A SURVIVOR, or I AM IN REMISSION. Don't give the 'C' word the power. It is a fear-based word that will keep you in a fearful state. Don't chatter endlessly about your cancer or your situation. You are expending valuable energy that can be used for your healing instead. Use empowering phrases such as, I AM GETTING HEALTHIER AND HEALTHIER EVERY DAY. Say kind and productive words about yourself and to others or don't speak at all. Repeat, I AM ENOUGH often, out loud or to yourself. Read your 'I am' list daily.

3. Laugh! Spend time with happy friends that support you and tell funny jokes and stories. Stay away from people who are negative or don't understand your path; they will bring you down. Watch funny movies. Happiness is contagious. Make it a point to laugh out loud. The physical vibration of laughing actually lowers your hormone and cortisol levels. Laughter also strengthens your immune system because it increases the production of antibodies in your saliva and in your bloodstream to stave off bacteria and viruses. I have heard miracle stories of people having spontaneous remission by just watching funny

movies all day and laughing. This also keeps your mind off your illness.

4. Help others and take the attention off yourself. Make a list of things you can do that would be of benefit to others and then start doing them and checking them off your list. Your inner happiness will start to grow quickly.

5. Walk in nature — especially in parks or forests. Breathe in the fresh oxygen and allow it to calm your nervous system and stir up your sense of wellbeing and happiness. Stop and look at the trees and truly notice them. Don't walk blindly through the woods — take your time and observe and be present. Mentally say your 'I am' list in your head. You can also do great forgiveness work as you walk. I would walk in the forest and repeat "I forgive you____". The act of forgiveness is very healing. I repeated it as I walked and absorbed the beauty around me. I did it until I felt that I had released my hurt and pain.

6. At night don't go to sleep until you are really tired. Don't lay there and think. If you're not tired, get up and get busy cleaning the house until you're really tired. Sweep the floor. Clean the toilet. Whatever it takes to get tired. Then get to bed and get yourself into a positive mental state by going through the list of things you are grateful for. (You can also do this in the morning.)

7. In your restful state, visualize your breasts surrounded by a HEALING WHITE LIGHT and ENERGY. See the white healing light swirl

around your breasts picking up all the cancerous cells and casting them off into the ether. Mentally state, 'Thank you for my perfect, healthy breasts.' Do this until there are no more dark cells left, and only the sparkling, white, perfect cells remain. Ten to twenty minutes is recommended or longer if you want.

8. Get help with releasing stuck emotions that are a roadblock to healing. Read 'The Emotion Code' by Dr. Bradley Nelson. I have met him and done his work and it is absolutely brilliant. Until then, observe your pain body when you feel any negative emotions arise. Separate yourself from them and become 'the watcher' of your pain body. Once you do this, you are no longer a part of it. You have separated yourself from it. For more information on this amazing technique read the wonderful book 'The Power of Now' by Eckhart Tolle.

9. Use the Ho'oponopono mantra prayer. I use it often and used it a lot during breast cancer. It is a traditional Hawaiian practice of reconciliation and forgiveness. Ho'oponopono is characterized in the Hawaiian dictionary as, 'Mental cleansing: family conferences in which relationships were set right (ho'oponopono) through prayer, discussion, confession, repentance, and mutual restitution and forgiveness'. The word ho'oponopono translates to 'causes things to move back in balance' or to 'make things right.' It's a very zen-like concept. (In native Hawaiian language, 'pono' means balance in life. Chanting this phrase over and

over is a powerful way to cleanse the body of long held guilt, shame, painful memories, bad will towards others, or negative thoughts.

There are four forces at work in this prayer: repentance, forgiveness, gratitude, and love. These are reflected in the four phrases that make up the prayer. The phrases, which you can repeat in any order, silently to yourself or out loud, are:

1. I'm sorry.
2. Please forgive me.
3. Thank you.
4. I love you.

The first step is about acceptance that all negativity starts within ourselves and we forgive ourselves for it. The second step is asking for forgiveness as a healing method that helps you move on in life. The third step is about gratitude and must be said repeatedly to bring in continuous positivity. The fourth step is about putting love into the world because it accelerates healing for ourselves and others. The four steps combined cleanse the heart, soul, mind and body.

Chapter 10

Eat To Stop Cancer Diet

I have included a slightly modified version of my daily nutritional protocol here so as not to overwhelm. For questions related to diet or more information please contact me at:

heidi@holisticbreastexpert.com

When I got breast cancer, I was already eating a very healthy diet so I didn't need to change that many things I was doing regarding my food intake, I just needed to refine it and become more strict. I eliminated all foods that weren't serving a higher purpose. That meant all sugar, including sugary fruits, alcohol, white bread, flour, pasta and potatoes, and all processed foods. Cancer feeds on sugar in our bodies and the last thing we want to do is feed it so it can grow bigger and stronger.

There are plenty of books on nutrition for combatting cancer so I won't repeat what is already widely available. What I can tell you, is everything I put in my mouth was considered a tool to get well. If I had any doubt about what I was putting in my mouth — I wouldn't eat it. It was as simple as that. I didn't care if I had to give up certain foods temporarily. To me, living was the most important thing and living meant using my diet as a powerful way to eliminate the cancer from my body, to heal it and to keep it from coming back. There are many ways to make vegetables and fruits taste delicious. They can be your friend if you let them! If you're not used to eating a clean diet, it will be an adjustment. Take steps every day to let go of old comforting eating habits and incorporate new additions from my list into your diet. Your body will thank you and you will get better much quicker.

My daily ritual:

- I drank fresh organic dark green vegetable juices throughout the day. I either went to a natural foods market or I juiced them myself. Most juices had a combination of spinach, kale, celery, and carrot, and often garlic and ginger.
- I drank wheat grass juice for a powerful antioxidant.
- I drank warm lemon water in the morning to cleanse my system.
- I eliminated all sugar from my diet.
- I eliminated all alcohol. Most alcohol is loaded with sugar.
- No red meat, pork or dairy products including eggs. (Processed meats, including hot dogs, salami and other cured meat products have been proven to be linked with higher rates of cancer.)
- I eliminated all white bread, white rice, white potatoes, pasta and processed foods. (Didn't eat

much anyway but definitely not during breast cancer)
- I drank 8 full glasses of water every day.
- I ate 80 percent raw foods, including a wide variety of vegetables, nuts and fresh citrus juices, especially grapefruit.
- I ate berries, which contain powerful antioxidants.
- I ate plenty of anti-cancer cruciferous vegetables including broccoli, cauliflower, kale, arugula and brussels sprouts—raw or very lightly steamed.
- I ate raw garlic every day.
- I drank green tea often — a powerful antioxidant.
- I ate fish and legumes for protein. (There is also plenty of protein in green vegetables.)
- I ate brown rice, oats and quinoa.

Supplements

- I took New Chapter turmeric force capsules as directed.
- I took Wobenzyme enzymes, a powerful anti-cancer formula that is advertised as an anti-inflammatory but is used for treating cancer in many alternative cancer clinics in the injectable form. (Check with your holistic practitioner for dosage and make sure to take them between meals or they will act as a digestive aid.)
- I took 4000 mg of Vitamin C capsules daily and Vitamin D.

- I took B complex, B12, B5 (panathonic acid) and B6 as directed.
- I took selenium and zinc and chlorophyll tablets as directed.
- I drank an ounce of wheatgrass juice every day.
- I drank the amazing anti cancer tea, Essiac or Fluoressence. (Almost the same formula. Fluorescence doesn't have the red clover ingredient as it is slightly estrogenic. Either one is good.)

A daily example

- Upon waking: Wobenzyme tablets on empty stomach.
- 4 ounces of warm water with a squeeze of fresh lemon juice for cleansing the system.
- Wait at least 15 minutes and then drink 4-6 ounces of Essiac tea on an empty stomach.
- Wait a half hour for breakfast: Whole grain sugar-free breakfast, for example, oatmeal, with fresh fruit, seeds, and nuts. Take vitamins.
- Fresh vegetable juice, with spinach, kale, celery, carrot, etc. and/or wheatgrass juice. Don't buy store bought. There is little fresh enzymatic action in juice after it sits for a few hours.
- Lunch: Dark green leafy salad filled with your favorite beans and peas and other veggies like carrot, beet, onion and fresh garlic. (be creative) Or an avocado sandwich on whole grain bread with lettuce, tomato. Side of carrots, broccoli and hummus.
- More dark green fresh vegetable juice.

- Snacks: Grab an apple, banana, or fresh berries. Dip carrots, celery, cucumbers, jicama, and peppers in hummus. Trail mix with nuts and dried fruit.
- Drinks: Hot or iced green tea with stevia.
- Dinner: Baked salmon with sweet potato, steamed or sautéed broccoli and veggies. Use Braggs Liquid Aminos as a seasoning, lemon and pepper.
- Before bed: 4-6 ounces of Essiac tea. Magnesium capsule for better sleep.

For more in-depth information on the eat to stop cancer diet, The Happy Healing project, guided meditations or mentoring programs, please contact me at heidi@holisticbreastexpert.com

Afterword

Once I made a decision to take control of my healing, everything shifted for me. I realized I had a lot more power over my healing than I was aware. I realized that by imagining my body to manufacture abundant healthy cells and operate in a cancer-free environment that it would take the orders and calibrate to be as I imagined. Research shows that just by visualizing a healthy body (and parts of it) every day for several minutes can alter physical cells and bring healing to that area.

Humans have much more ability to heal themselves than we give them credit for. Doctors focus on the cure. Our bodies focus on healing. We can shift matter inside our bodies when we focus our mind into dynamic willpower. This willpower alters and compiles the energetic frequency inside of us so that healing can take place. There is nothing mystical about how this happens. It is the same intelligence that organizes and balances all the functions of the body every second of the day. It keeps our heart pumping two gallons of blood every day. Dr. Joe Dispenza states: "your thoughts condition your mind and your feelings condition your body. And when you have mind and body working together, you have the power of the universe behind you."

Every day I imagined myself as perfectly healthy. I had the surgery and the lump was gone. I had my lymph nodes checked to see if it had spread and it hadn't. So I knew that the cancer was gone from my body. I saw myself as completely healed.

I didn't have belief anymore, I just knew.

I didn't entertain the word remission at all. Remission infers that the cancer cells are just laying dormant 'sleeping' somewhere and if we're not careful they will wake up and come back again! Forget that. I never said that word. If anyone asked me if I was in remission I would say: "No — the cancer is gone!"

I imagined my breast healthy and vibrant with all the cells perfect and operating at their highest capacity. I saw it over and over — every day, when I woke up and when I went to bed and throughout the day.

Thoughts have a frequency and if enough of our thoughts surrounding our illness shift over to the positive, we get well.

Every day I affirmed how grateful I was. I went through my gratitude list and once I had said thank you several times, I would feel my emotional vibration shift and elevate. I used the ho'opono'ono mantra throughout my day.

I would also meditate for 20 minutes or longer and elevate my consciousness to a more calm and focused place. Towards the end of the meditation when I was in an elevated meditative state, I saw my body perfectly healthy and whole and protected by my high power. I would stay in that space and focus on the shift inside my body as I saw myself well in the quantum field of consciousness. I would end the meditation with: "Thank you for my perfect health".

I got to THE KNOWING place.

If you don't have total faith that you can get well — you can't. If you don't believe you have the power to heal yourself — you won't.

If you continuously entertain thoughts of your cancer, bad health, struggle, death, etc, then it will be much harder to get well. You need to be firmly planted in your conviction.

Every single day.

At times it feels like work. But, it's good work. At times, you doubt yourself and feel like nothing's happening. But, if you push aside the small negative voice that pops in to steal your joy enough times, it will shut up.

Every day I was hyper-focused on all things healing and for my highest good. Meditation, yoga, healthy raw foods, fresh green juices, yoga, walking, but most importantly, a new positive mindset.

People around me started to talk. What's up with Heidi? Why is she so happy? Doesn't she have cancer?

And if they asked me, I would say: "I used to have it, but not anymore."

About the Author

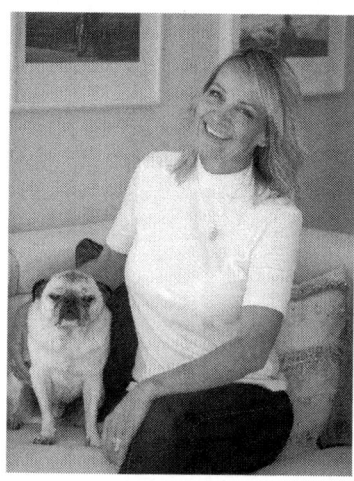

Heidi Sorensen is a counselor, coach and health mentor for women with breast cancer and other health-related issues. She is also a certified mindfulness meditation teacher and has been practicing Kriya Yoga meditation since she was 19 years old.

Heidi divides her time between Southern California and Vancouver, B.C. Canada where she works as a health mentor and writer. She is a former actor, singer and model and knows a thing or two about breasts as she was also Miss July, 1981 for Playboy Magazine. Since then, she has advocated for the rights of girls and women through her own non-profit society and with The Ending Violence Association of Canada, WeSolve People 2 People conferences in association with the U.S. Department of Defense and other international organizations, including World Vision. Heidi is also a public speaker on the topic of using mind-set for healing.

Heidi has a strong passion for all things wind and ocean. Her daughter is pure joy and laughter and the love of her life and her 19 year old pug, Edward, keeps her on her toes. She gathers wisdom from trees and each day is much more exhilarating with a nice cup of tea.

For questions or inquiries related to public speaking, Heidi can be reached by email at: heidi@holisticbreastexpert.com or you can visit her website at holisticbreastexpert.com

Printed in Great Britain
by Amazon